STOP
MASTURBATING
AND
START LIVING

How to go from fappy to happy and overcome any vice or addiction

JOSEPH FAN, ESQ.

ISBN10: 0-9987343-0-6

ISBN13: 978-0-9987343-0-9

Cover design by: Mandy Cat Kitana

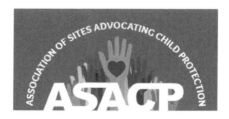

A portion of the proceeds of this book will be donated to Association of Sites Advocating Child Protection (ASACP) Foundation, a 501(c)(3) nonprofit charitable organization. The ASACP Foundation operates the ASACP child exploitation reporting tipline, the Restricted To Adults - RTA Website Label, and provides educational and technological resources for anyone wanting to better protect children online. (www.asacp.org)

To the love of my life, Julia

CONTENTS

Foreword

Before we begin, let's get something important out of the way—masturbation, as used in this book, is a metaphor for any vice. The principles in this book can be applied to anything from drinking too much alcohol, watching too many dumb videos online, to biting your fingernails. So you just picked up a book that will help you overcome self-sabotage. Are you excited? You should be! Ok, let's start...

If you didn't get it by the title, this is a book about masturbation and how to either stop doing it or keep it under control so your life is not negatively affected by it. This book is for anyone who wants to stop masturbating and is ready to take back their life. It is also for anyone who wants to understand what someone else who is trying to stop masturbating is going through. Masturbation does not have to be taboo. This is a serious subject, a serious addiction for some, that you may be dealing with hands-on (as you will see, all the puns in this book are intended).

It is also noteworthy to mention that I am speaking as a heterosexual male about my experience of male masturbation.

Now that is out of the way, my name is Joseph Fan. I was a chronic masturbator for most of my life. What I mean by that is I have masturbated, on average, an hour every day, between ages 7 and 27 (at the time of the publishing of this book, I am 30), with the exception of three separate weeks at a summer sleep-away camp when I was 15, a one-month no-masturbation streak when I was 19, and three eight-day trips to Burning Man. I have had a few two or three day masturbation-free streaks, but because I also had probably a greater number of three or four hour weekend fap-fests,[1] the time I spent masturbating roughly averages out to about one hour a day. My masturbation routine had remained mostly the same throughout life. Something along the lines of: wake up, go to

---

[1] Fap is slang for masturbation. It comes from the sound that is made when masturbation is taking place.

school/work, run home, go to my room, turn on music, put on headphones, and masturbate to pornography. Rinse and repeat.

At 20 years of masturbating an hour a day, subtracting the 63 confirmed masturbation-free days, I estimate I have masturbated 7,237 hours in my 20 years of masturbation. That is 301.5 days straight, give or take a few days – almost one full year of my life shot into a wad of tissues.

Some of you may be shocked; some of you may relate; and some of you have surpassed me threefold. But regardless, as a first exercise, you should estimate how much time you have spent masturbating. This can be a real eye opener when you actually do the math.

Since I have stopped chronically masturbating, I have amazed myself with the things I have accomplished. I have developed closer relationships to my friends and family. I proposed to my then girlfriend (now wife) with a one thousand person flash mob at Daybreaker.[2] I have taken up standup comedy and jujitsu. I play a lot more ice hockey. I founded a nonprofit organization to end street harassment and serve as the general counsel for that organization. I became a life coach and a fashion coach. I started a career as a real estate broker and started my own real estate firm. Even writing this book would have been time spent masturbating.

---

[2] Daybreaker is a sober, early-morning dance party that takes place around the world. Find out more about them at www.daybreaker.com.

I am not trying to sell you a magic pill – everything you need in order to stop masturbating is already at your disposal. It may seem impossible because refraining from masturbating can take a lot of self-control, energy, and time, but look back on your life and notice all the things you've overcome using your self-control, energy, and time – you've got this! An unfortunate reality about our lives is that time is a non-renewable resource, and we will never get back any time wasted. Fortunately, we can control what we do with the rest of the time we have left.

Replace masturbation with whatever it is you want to do instead! Read on to learn how!

<u>Why I wrote this book</u>

I wrote this book as much for myself as for you, dear reader. Have you ever been told that masturbation leads to blindness or causes you to grow hair on your palms, and every time you masturbate a puppy dies? If those were the only side effects, masturbation would not be so bad.

I have experienced firsthand the monster that pornography and chronic masturbation has turned me into. It has brought out the worst in me. I also experienced the gifts that come with harnessing the power and energy the body and mind naturally exudes and applying them to things that actually matter to me.

When we are born, we start off as a blank slate. Our experiences make us who we are. Pornography adds to that slate. Masturbation adds to that slate. If we spend a big chunk of our lives (for example, almost one-twentieth, as I have) in that masturbation mindset, it becomes ingrained in us.

Though I give a few practical tips, this book is predominantly about mindset. We are all wired differently, and what works for me might not work for you. If something works for you, run with it! My hope is that by reading this, you will be able to actively and fully make the choice to stop masturbating and grab *life* by the balls

instead.

Why do you want to stop?

Honestly, without lying to yourself, why do you really want to stop masturbating and watching pornography? Is it because of social stigma? Religion? Your partner? Do you actually want to stop?

I only ask these initial questions because if you want to stop for any reason other than because YOU want to stop, then it is the wrong reason. Be clear that you and only you should be the driving factor behind your decisions and actions.

There is nothing inherently bad about

masturbation and/or pornography.

Masturbation can be healthy even if you do it every day, multiple times a day. It is when it gets in the way of you being the person that you want to be that it becomes a problem. If you do not consider it a waste of your time, it excites, energizes, and motivates you, and contributes to your life, then by all means, why stop? Why did you even pick up this book?

If you think about it, that's actually pretty funny – you CAN CHOOSE to let masturbation and/or pornography motivate and inspire you.

The beauty of being alive and free is that you have choice. Remember, you can literally do anything you want. Yes, there are consequences to your actions, but YOU CAN LITERALLY DO ANYTHING YOU WANT. You can choose and take responsibility for your choices. You MUST CHOOSE.

You can choose to, or choose not to, but the power is in your choice. Be conscious in your choice.

Are you sure you want to close those fifty-eight tabs?

Are you sure you want to permanently delete that hidden folder on your hard drive?

Are you sure you are ready to free up some time to create an awesome life surrounded by friends and family, being healthy, creating wealth, and loving your life?

YES! ... or NO! Choose consciously!

Either answer is perfect, so long as you recognize you have the choice and you consciously made that choice.

Use this in every area of your life, and I promise you will experience so much power that stopping masturbating will be such an easy obstacle to overcome, you will not believe it was ever even a problem.

How do you feel after masturbating?

I know you feel great while masturbating, but in those moments after, how do you feel?

Really live with this.

Personally, I feel ashamed, regretful, tired, de-motivated. Ashamed at what I watched or imagined while masturbating. Regretful of the time I wasted. Physically and mentally tired from the exercise itself. Unmotivated to do anything else, with shame, regret, and fatigue hanging over me. You might feel this way, you might not.

The next time you are going to masturbate, ask

yourself: Knowing how you are going to feel afterwards, do you want to go forward with this?

The easiest way to actually do this is to have some sort of reminder, either a sticker on your computer, or a bracelet on your wrist to symbolize your new commitment.

Are you addicted?

Masturbation was like the friend I never had who was always there for me. Certainly, it has helped me through some tough times, like when I was bullied and beaten up in middle school and high school for having acne, being scrawny and short, Asian, and/or poor. When I had social anxiety and would shake when I spoke to girls. It was stress relief when I was at law school in a competitive and close-minded environment. I knew I could always go home and at least *I* would fuck myself.

However, at some point, my acne cleared up. I started getting fit and got a little taller. I started making money. I developed great social skills that earned me more friends than I could count and allowed me to date beautiful women. (I never did stop being Asian though).

I thought finding a girlfriend would cure me. It did not. And it wasn't like I was not having sex – I was having a lot of it. However, I was masturbating in addition to the sex. Eventually, things got so bad that I preferred masturbation to sex. I was addicted to masturbation.

Is your masturbation habit an addiction? Are you addicted to masturbation and/or pornography? Does it stop you from fully enjoying your life?

What do you think about in the five minutes of post-climax clarity?

Ah, the five minutes of clarity after you climax and you are no longer distracted by your sexual urges. Wouldn't it be great if we could just live full-time in this period? A time when everything just makes sense. And you think to yourself – If you just put as much effort into doing the things you love, you would be a "better" person.

And then you look down and feel the sense of regret. At this point, you may delete your hard drive of porn, trash your magazines, begin to

18

reformat your faptop (a laptop full of viruses used solely for the purposes of storing and watching porn). And then you wonder... What did I just watch? Where did the day go? What did I accomplish? I think I am going to take a nap. Well, tomorrow is a new day (but we both know it is not really)! And then it begins again. You undo the delete, are glad you didn't delete the history in your web browser, and get back to your masturbation-filled existence.

Technology is amazing. Today, humans have the entirety of knowledge at their fingertips. We can send messages instantly across the world. We can fly in iron birds across oceans. But technology comes at a price.

We also have lifelike masturbation sleeves, sex dolls, and powerful vibrating massage wands. We have the ability to look up any person who has ever been naked in front of a camera and see them instantly. There is virtual reality porn. Were we meant to have this gluttony?

What if you don't stop?

If the cliché quote, "The definition of insanity is doing the same thing over and over and expecting different results," holds true, if you do nothing, you will continue to dedicate a chunk of your life to masturbation and your life will continue on the path it is currently on with even more masturbation under your belt.

How is your life right now? Is it everything you dreamed it would be? Could it be even better? What would one uninterrupted year of intense focus and concentration help you accomplish?

What are you supposed to do instead?

What are you supposed to do with all that pent-up sexual energy? USE IT!

What do you enjoy doing? Do that instead. Love whoever you are with. Make love to your partner(s). Enjoy being alive. Dance. Eat good food. Get in touch with your spirituality. Save the rainforests. Or dolphins. Go to the gym. Read a book. Write a book. Start a business.

Get this: instead of one-way interactions through a computer screen, you can develop real connections with actual people.

This is what the good life looks like – living with the fullest love, wealth, health, and happiness.

How can you do this?

Imagine that from this moment on, every time you masturbated, a finger was cut off. Which finger would you be down to before you'd consider stopping? If you were like me and had to move onto the toes, then you can see how serious of a problem this is.

You can do this, and I know you can. Here is an illustration of why I am so sure: think about the person that means the most to you in this world. Now imagine there is a gun aimed at this person's head that will go off if you masturbated.

I wouldn't even have to finish that sentence for you to understand that you would be "cured." But that is not the case. No one has your hand on a butcher's block or your loved one at gunpoint. But what if you lived as though masturbating caused life-altering consequences like that? I am not suggesting that you buy a guillotine or hire someone to kidnap your loved one. But in order to play this game with intensity and feel some pain, why not put a deterrent in place where if you masturbate, you have to donate $100 to the politician you disagree with most? Or choose your most valuable possession and pledge it to a cause you do not believe in? You can even get an accountability buddy to make sure you follow through. You get the idea – actually put something you care about on the line.

Well, your life is on the line, isn't it? Isn't that why you picked up this book? Because there are things you want to accomplish that you haven't even started? Seriously, this is your life we're talking about.

On the other side of the coin, how is that any way to live life, having constant anxiety knowing that in a moment of weakness, there will be a major consequence?

There are practical solutions to forcibly prevent masturbation. Medication, chastity devices, hiring someone to follow you around everywhere you go to punch you in the face every time you are about to masturbate. There are also less extreme solutions, such as using apps that block pornography sites. But you might just find a way to bypass them. Guilt as a de-motivator is also effective for some people. It is true, that the people in the pornographic films are people's parents, siblings, and children, but these are just not pleasant things to think about and they don't really leave you inspired and motivated to harness that energy and excitement to do something else.

Here is the formula to stop masturbating and reclaim your life:

Face yourself in the mirror.

Think back to the last time you masturbated. What were you watching? What were you thinking? Where were you? How did you do it? Be descriptive. How did you feel while doing it? How did you feel after? Write this down. Do not hold anything back.

It will help seeing your own handwriting. Read it to yourself in the mirror. There is something very powerful about seeing ourselves being authentic.

Declare to yourself, "Today is day one of my masturbation-free diet. My new life will be amazing because I am going to use the time, energy and motivation to live the good life!"

Declare your intention publically.

Now that you've faced your harshest and most important critic (yourself!), announce to everyone else in your life that you will stop masturbating and how much time you've wasted doing it in the past. Own it!

There is something very powerful in being vulnerable with people. Once your cards are on the table, there's nothing left to hide. You can finally be yourself. This is pure freedom.

Announcing this to the world will ensure you follow through because now you can ask people to hold you accountable.

Join a community.

Though this book is titled *Stop Masturbating and Start Living*, it is not associated with NoFap, a secular porn addiction and masturbation recovery community (they have a subreddit).

This community is amazing and full of people going through the same thing as you. There are also many religious groups that hold similar weekly meetups. Find a community that works for you. When you have a community that contributes to you and allows you to contribute to them, you'll be less likely to give it all up for a moment of self-induced short term pleasure.

Make it a game.

Aren't games more fun than chores? Don't see this as something dull that you don't want to do. It is not about the number of days straight that you have gone without masturbating, though you can use that as a measure.

Treat it as a challenge that will ensure that your

life gets better. The reward is that you get to pursue something you love or that you've always wanted to do.

Remember, it is about what you get to do instead of masturbating – what you get to accomplish! Don't focus on <u>not</u> masturbating – focus on the new things you are taking on instead. The positive is always more inspiring and powerful.

Meditate.

I used to have trouble meditating. I always thought I was doing it wrong and never really got anything out of it. But meditation does not have to be like what you see on TV or what you imagine a Buddhist monk does while sitting motionless and silent in a temple.

The purpose of meditating is to recenter yourself. This will soothe your temptations so you can do the things that really matter to you.

When I meditate, I sit or stand upright with my eyes closed and I breathe normally. I imagine that I am alone in space, surrounded by all the flowing energy of the universe. With each inhaling breath, I breathe in all the possibilities of things that I can do. With each exhaling breath, I breathe out everything else. I concentrate on that, and if I lose concentration, no worries – I just begin again. The beauty of this meditation is that you don't have to force anything – your mind will take care of everything.

Notice I did not put a time limit. That is because

meditation can take as long or as short as you need. It can take place at the office during the time you would use for a cigarette break. It can be when you wake up with morning wood. It could be in three seconds on a crowded train car.

In our context, we are using it to stop doing one thing and direct that energy, focus, motivation, and time to other things that are important to us. Do this meditation consistently, and you will see that after some time, only the latter part of our purpose will be there.

The secret

Malcolm Gladwell popularized the 10,000 Hour Theory – 10,000 hours of "deliberate practice" would make someone world-class in that field. Whether or not this theory is true, I submit that 10,000 hours of doing anything will make you at least really, really good at it.

What could you have accomplished in all that time you spent masturbating? Some of you reading could have found the cure for cancer. Others could have volunteered and made a difference in other people's lives. We could have created a shitload of art. Maybe we could have spent more time with family and friends; learned a language or multiple languages fluently; became an expert at a craft or sport; or learned how to play an instrument.

Instead of the above accomplishments, what I have to show for my time is a vast mental database of pornstar names, the best websites for watching specific types of porn, different types of degrading sex acts, and abbreviations for various porn terminology. And as I got tired of vanilla pornography, I sought out more extreme gonzo hardcore porn.

Ask anyone whether, if they could magically trade all their hours masturbating for hours training for the Olympics, creating a successful business, or getting really good at something else, would they? The likely answer is yes; they would trade in those short-term gratifications.

Here is the secret you've been waiting for and have known all along: there is still time! You could be the person you want to be. The best time to start something is ten years ago – the second best time is right now. The next time you feel like masturbating, actively choose not to and dedicate that time to doing whatever activity you've chosen to get really good at.

I could have written a much longer and thicker book so that you would feel like you got your money's worth, but I've said everything I needed to say. The whole point of this book being concise is for it to be read in the amount of time it would take to masturbate. So look – you've had your first victory! You read my book instead of masturbating!

Remember that these are only words on paper. Reading this book will make no difference without action. It is up to you to implement this in your life. So stop masturbating and start living!

Postscript

By now, you've probably realized that this book is not just about how to stop masturbating (especially since the first sentence in the book tells you this). It's about taking control of your life. Everyone has their own vices – for me, it was masturbation. But the lessons in this book can be applied to any vice in your life, from drinking to procrastination to emotional eating. Replace the word "masturbation" with the thing(s) preventing you from reaching your full potential and preventing you from doing all the things you want to in life. Stop ____ing and START LIVING!

<u>Acknowledgements</u>

First and foremost, Julia, my wife, my way better half, my moral compass, I love you more than words can ever even begin to... Thank you for being such an amazing and understanding partner in crime and for all your encouragement.

Thank you Mom and Dad for always knocking before coming in when I lived under your roof and letting me do my own laundry. I hope this book is never translated into Chinese.

My uncle Lun Chang, you showed me such strength during your battle with cancer and I will take that with me throughout my life.

Susan and David, my wonderful in-laws, mentors, and white parents I never had but always wanted, I love you. Your believing in me has made me believe in myself more than I have ever believed in anyone else ever.

Thank you Mandy Cat Kitana for all your support, love, and your beautiful cover art. Your artistic vision is unmatched and you have no idea how much you have inspired me.

My brother Gearóid, thank you for all the edits you made on the book design.

My literary agent and friend, Alex Rubin, thank you for all your guidance in making this book a reality.

My StartingBloc family, I am still truly touched at the outpour of advice from all the accomplished authors and speakers who took the time to talk to me and take me seriously.

The Daybreaker Community, especially Eli, Radha, Molly, and Elliot, your early morning sober dance parties have changed my life and gave me the courage to move forward with this book.

The NoFap community, I have always been a lurker, but know that you have helped me through more hard times than I can count.

Tim and The Association of Sites Advocating Child Protection (ASACP), thank you for all the important work you do and thank you for allowing me to make this project bigger than myself.

Last but not least, this book would not be possible without all the hardworking pornstars and porn companies out there!

There are many others, you know who you are...

Sorry I am not sorry to anyone I have offended with the publication of this book.

Thank You

Thank YOU for reading my book. I truly hope it has helped you the same way putting down all these words on paper helped me. If you have a second, please follow me on all those social media platforms everyone is always talking about:

Facebook, YouTube, Instagram: Exchange Defeat For Victory

Twitter: @exchangedefeat

If you ever need to reach me, you can email me at stopmasturbatingandstartliving@gmail.com.

The official website for this book:

www.StopMasturbatingAndStartLiving.com

If this book has helped you, I would be forever grateful if you could leave a review on Amazon.

Made in the USA
Monee, IL
12 November 2020